THE TAO
OF DYING

Library of Congress Catalog Card Number 94-69-243
ISBN-09628363-9-7

THE TAO
OF DYING

written by
Doug Smith

photographs by
Marilu Pittman

CARING
PUBLISHING

519 C Street, NE, Stanton Park, Washington, DC 20002-5809

Introduction

The Tao Te Ching was written about 2,500 years ago by a man named Lao Tzu. The book was intended as a guide for living a meaningful life. Much of the book also seems quite appropriate for assisting in the facilitation of a meaningful death. It is this appropriateness that inspires the following paraphrase of the Tao Te Ching, paraphrased to meet the needs and the desires of the terminally ill.

Addressing the needs and the desires of the terminally ill in recent times has been strongly influenced by the ever-expanding hospice movement with its emphasis on the concept of palliation. This concept can be defined simply as caring for people without trying to change or cure them. This definition of palliation closely parallels the Tao Te Ching's central concept of *wei wu wei*, literally translated as doing by not doing. Both of these concepts, palliation and *wei wu wei*, affirm a way of interacting that is characterized by accepting people, things, and processes for what they are without trying to manipulate, alter, or control them. These concepts inspire the thoughts of this book.

Inspiration for this book also comes from writings and

research in the field of thanatology. Much of the recent writings and research in that field center around improving the quality of the dying person's environment, aiming for a "good" death. This kind of thinking comes from well-seasoned theories such as Phillippe Aries' theory of a "tamed" death and Avery Weisman's theory of an "appropriate" death, as well as my own developing theory of a "healthy" death. All these theories agree on common descriptions of the ideal environment for the dying: providing the dying with as much control as possible, allowing for many opportunities for reminiscense, laughter, expressions of anger and sadness, the experience of touching and being touched, and explorations of spirituality, as well as accepting whatever style of coping the dying person chooses to exercise — in short, allowing the dying to think, do, or be whatever the dying want to think, do, or be.

Finally, the most profound inspiration for this book comes from the dying themselves. That inspiration is lovingly captured in the touching photographs of Marilu Pittman. Her photographs show us that it is the dying themselves who enliven within their caregivers an awe that can only manifest itself in caring without trying to change or cure, respecting without limiting that respect, allowing without ever needing to control. That is true palliation. That is true *wei wu wei.*

Dedication

For my father, Bill
For my brother, Dean
For my daughter, Kristin

For all those who continue
to teach us that our times together
will always be so very brief.
We also need to make them very precious.

~ Doug Smith

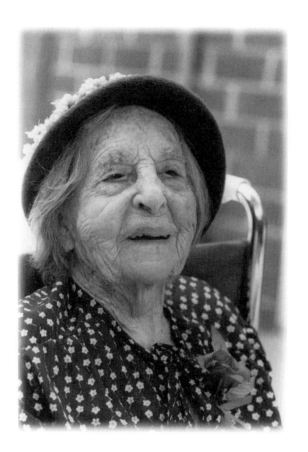

What-has-been has been.
What-is is.
What-will-be will be.

What-will-be comes from what-is.
What-is comes from what-has-been.

Why do we argue with what-has-been?
Why do we fight with what-is?
Why do we try to control what-will-be?

The practice of allowing reveals what is true.
The practice of trying to control hides what is true.

Your dying and my dying are the same in meaning.
Yet all manifestations will always be different.
Realize the common meaning.
Respect the many manifestations.

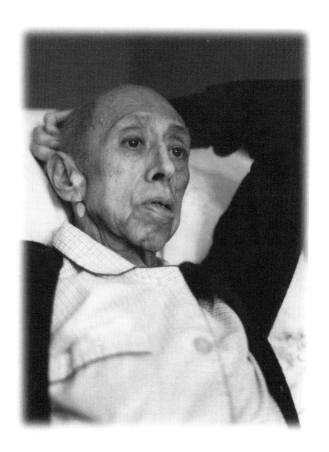

When we label some deaths right,
other deaths become wrong.
When we label some deaths good,
other deaths become bad.

Living and dying create each other.
The easy way and the difficult way are interdependent.
The long life and the short life are relative.
The first days and the last days accompany each other.

Therefore, the true caregiver of the dying
does all that needs to be done without asserting herself,
and says all that needs to be said without saying anything.
Things happen, and she allows them to happen;
Things fail to happen, and she allows them to fail to happen.
She is always there,
but it is as though she is not there.
She realizes that she does nothing,
yet all that needs to be done is done.

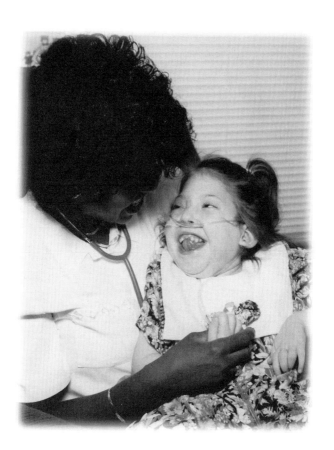

If you overvalue living,
    dying becomes valueless.
    If you invest everything in what is now,
    what is yet to come has been stolen from you.

    The caregiver of the dying cares
    by not trying to change or cure.
    In allowing for that which seems to be unallowable,
    in tolerating that which appears to be intolerable,
    and in accepting that which looks like it is unacceptable,
    the caregiver of the dying is a true giver of care.

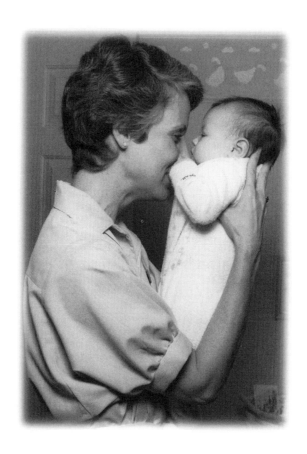

The process of dying is nothing out of the ordinary.
The moment of death is a single point on a circle.
The point of death is indistinguishable from
the point of birth.

Birth and death are inseparable.
Living and dying are inseparable.
Birth welcomes death.
Death welcomes birth.

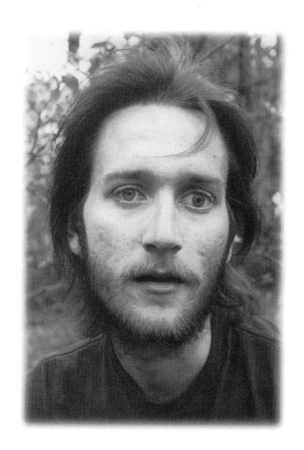

The process of dying does not favor anyone.
It visits men and women, black and white, good and bad.
The process of dying does not practice prejudice
of any kind.

Death erases meaning.
Yet without death there can be no meaning.

Try to grasp hold of death,
and you will see there is nothing to grasp.
The process of dying has a hold on you.

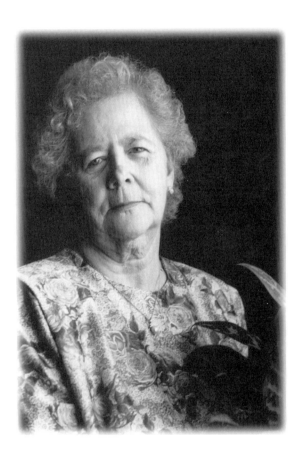

The caregiver's practice of allowing:
   it does nothing and therefore partakes in everything.
   The practice of allowing facilitates
   the past, the present, and the future.

   By not controlling,
   you are welcomed into the limitless.

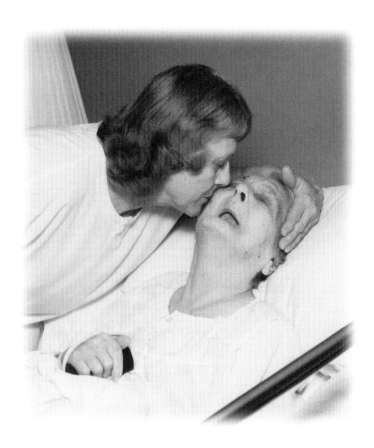

The caregiver of the dying partakes in the limitless.
She partakes in the limitless
because she leaves no trace of her presence.
Because she does not control,
the caregiver of the dying partakes in the limitless.

Because nothing needs to be accomplished,
all is accomplished that needs to be.

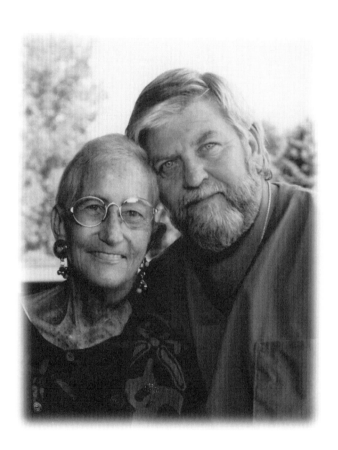

The caregiver of the dying is like water.
He does not wish to be in high places.
He chooses to recede to the low places.

His emotions value the emotions of others.
His thoughts value the thoughts of others.
His words value the words of others.
His actions value the actions of others.
Therefore, all is accomplished that needs
to be accomplished.

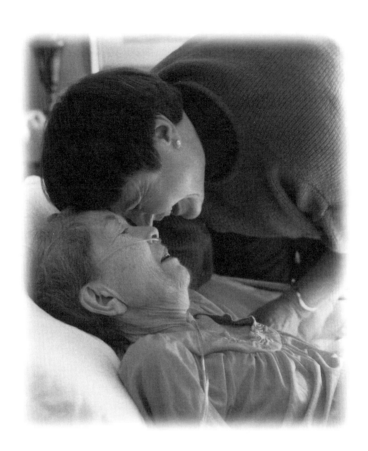

To spend all that you have
is to have nothing left.
To have only good moments
is the same as having only bad moments.
To think that you know everything
is to cheat yourself from learning anything.
Learn your limits,
and you will partake in the limitless.

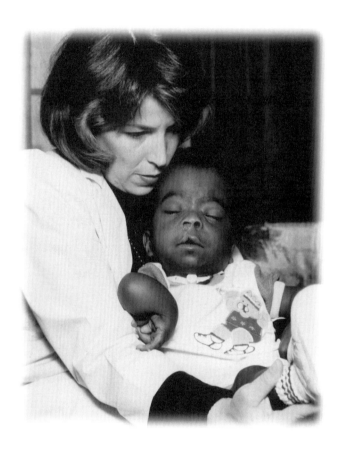

Can you forget all of your agendas so that you can
become a part of the only agenda?
Can you become like a newborn, ready to learn
and ready to grow with every new happening?
Can you forget about all of your past in order
to be fully present?
Can you love without trying to control?
Can you stop working so that you can play along?
Can you do all that needs to be done
without doing anything?

The virtue that others see in you is proportionate
to the virtue that you see in others.

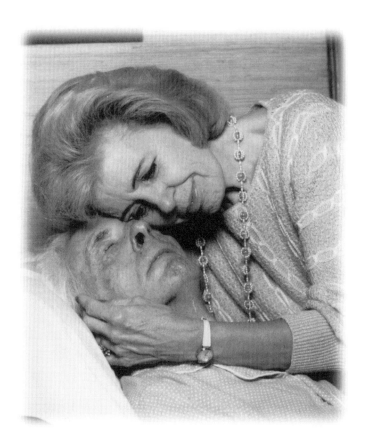

Many spokes can make a wheel strong.
Yet the wheel serves no purpose at all without
the center hole.

Colorfully painted clay can make a pretty pot.
Yet the pot serves no purpose at all if there
is no emptiness within.

We may use the finest woods to construct a house.
Yet the house serves no purpose at all without
any inner space.

We may try as hard as we may.
Yet it is in not trying that we serve a purpose.

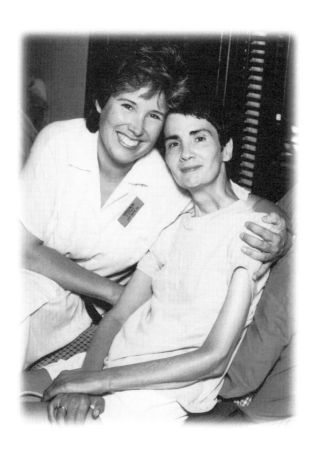

Too many colors confuse the eyes.
Too many sounds confuse the ears.
Too many flavors confuse the taste buds.
Too many thoughts confuse the mind.
Too many desires confuse the will.

The caregiver of the dying has knowledge
of the complex world.
Yet the caregiver relies upon the simple things.

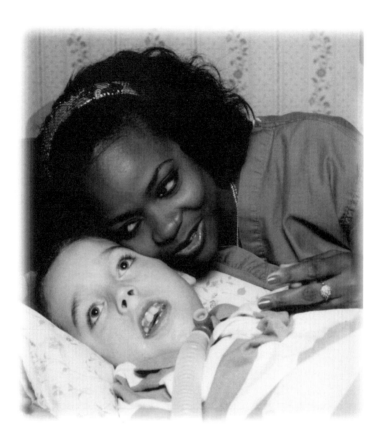

Be not concerned when being praised or blamed.
Both praise and blame can be heavy burdens.

If you take praise for doing one thing,
you will be worried if you are not praised
for the next thing.
If you take blame for doing one thing,
you will worry over receiving blame
for the next thing.

The taking of too much praise causes one
to inflate the self.
The taking of too much blame causes one
to deflate the self.

She who forgets about herself,
not caring about inflation or deflation of herself,
is fully present for other selves.

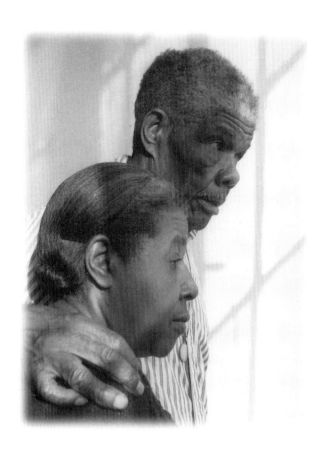

Look for the invisible.
Listen to the inaudible.
Touch the immaterial.

In experiencing nothing,
the caregiver of the dying experiences
everything imaginable.
In being nothing,
the caregiver of the dying
becomes everything imaginable.

Controlling makes everything into nothing.
Allowing makes nothing into everything.

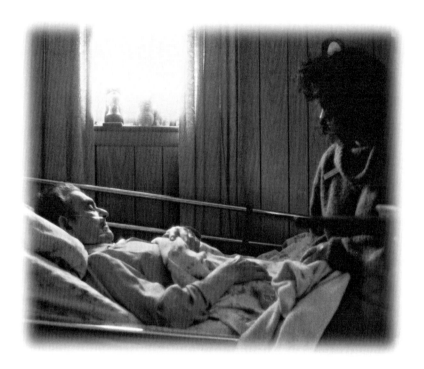

The great teachers of the past cannot be labeled,
defined, or even remotely described.

Like the wind, their power was felt
but could not be delineated.
Like the uncarved block of wood,
their potential was inexhaustible.
Like water, they could grow the tallest trees or form
the deepest valleys or merely watch the fishes play.

So, the caregiver of the dying waits,
waiting for her task to be set.

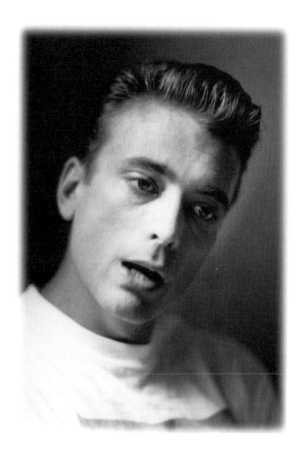

Empty your mind of all preconceived ideas.

Be coming home wherever you are.

Allow everyone to be a part of the homecoming.

Every individual travels the journey from birth to death.

No matter how rugged the journey,

the journey's end allows for the ruggedness to cease.

If you do not fully comprehend that the journey must end,

you will experience a journey of painful dissolution.

In selflessness, realize that there is no pain in dissolution.

There is only pain in hanging on.

So let go.

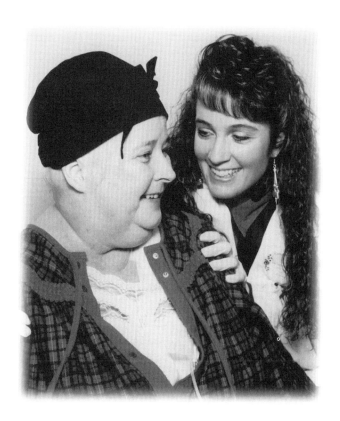

When the caregiver allows a death
to take its natural course,
her presence is hardly known at all.
A lesser caregiver is one who is loved and praised.
An even lesser caregiver is one who is feared.
The worst caregiver is one who is despised.

It is when the caregiver does not trust others
that others do not trust her.

The caregiver of the dying does not talk; she acts.
She acts in such a way that no credit goes to her.
When all has been finished in the right way,
she receives no credit, and no credit is deserved.

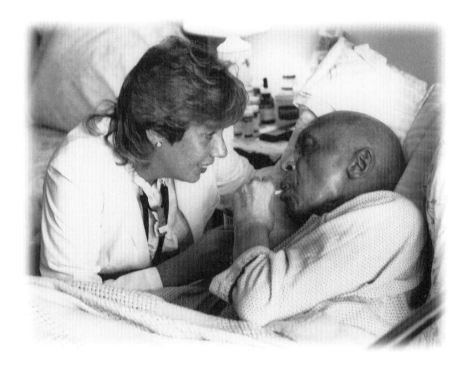

When caregivers lose the way,
goodness and righteousness come to the fore.
When caregivers forget
about the world's natural intelligence,
cleverness and wisdom rear their ugly heads.
When caregivers assert their ways,
peace is lost, a battle begins, turmoil reigns.

The way of caregiving is the way of allowing.
Step back to find the way.

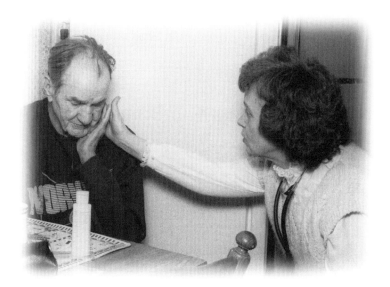

Rid the world of philosophers and theorists.
Throw out all the research studies.
Then the importance of people will come to the fore.

Abandon your control,
and the dying will find an abundance of choices.
Abandon your past experiences,
and the dying will recognize beauty
in both the present and future.
Abandon your religion,
and the dying will discover their own spirituality.

Empty yourself,
and the world will be full.

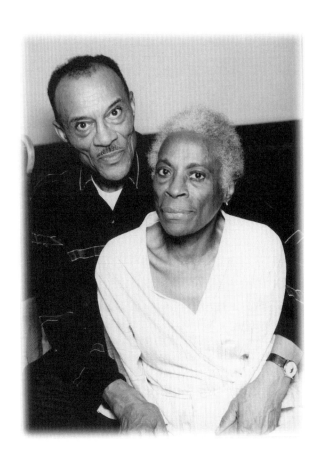

To try to change or cure death is complete foolishness.
To simply care for the dying
is the ultimate accomplishment.
Yet it is an accomplishment that deserves no merit.

Not trying to reach for what is beyond reach,
the caregiver enjoys his role.
Not trying to achieve what cannot be achieved,
the caregiver enjoys his role.
Not trying to control what cannot be controlled,
the caregiver enjoys his role.

Other people claim to have the light,
while he claims to be in the dark.
Other people claim to be on top of things,
while he claims to be at the bottom.
Other people claim to be at the forefront,
while he comes up from behind.

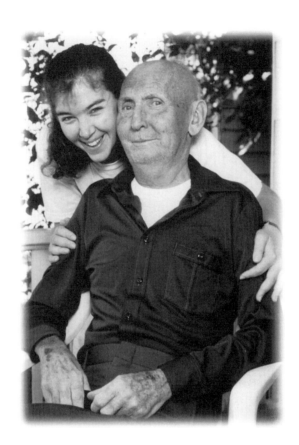

In maintaining an attitude of allowing,
the caregiver participates in the mystery of creation.

The mystery of endings comes
with the mystery of beginnings.
The caregiver accepts and respects the mystery of both.

Allowing for the mystery, the caregiver becomes
a part of the mystery.

The mystery is around her.
The mystery is within her.
Together, she and the mystery smile.

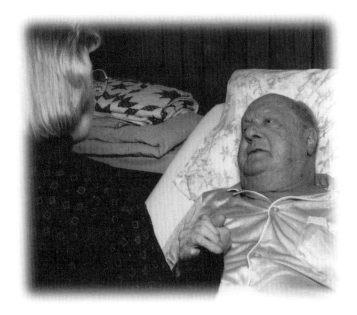

The agitated will eventually receive calm,
and the painful will eventually find comfort,
and the exhausted will eventually find rest.
The unfinished business will eventually need no resolution.

So the caregiver of the dying gives herself to the process
as a model for friends and family.
Remaining in the shadows,
she gives light to all around her.
Remaining in passivity,
she becomes an active agent.
Allowing the process to occur,
she has no need to control anything.

By being a servant,
she has become the Master.

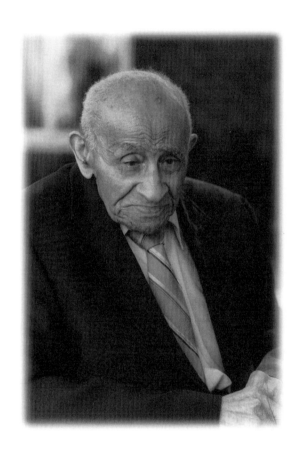

The best things can be communicated without
the use of words.
All the commotion runs its course.
Disruptions come to their own conclusion.
So, keep quiet!
Words mean so much less than actions,
and the best action is no action at all.

If you do what is right,
you will see what is right be done.
If you do what is good,
you will see what is good be done.
If you forget what is right and good,
you will see what is right and good be forgotten.

Power comes to those who know how to allow
for the giving of power.
Benefits come to those who know how to allow
for the giving of benefits.
Power is lost and benefits are non-existent
for those who are trying to grasp at them.

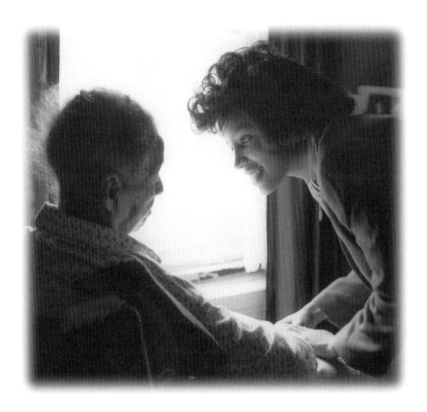

Boast about yourself,

and you will find yourself ashamed.

Give yourself prominence,

and you will be humbled.

Praise yourself,

and watch how you will be degraded.

Make yourself important,

and you will become embarrassed.

Your bragging brings only your humiliation.

Simply allow the dying person freedom,

and you will find yourself giving credit

where credit is due.

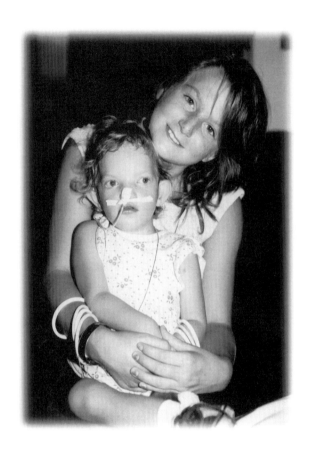

The mystery of beginnings and endings
is beyond description.
Foolish people limit the mystery
through words and concepts.
We must merely allow for the mystery.

There is mystery in birth.
There is mystery in death.
Every individual is a mystery.
The whole world is a mystery.

We must allow for the mystery.
We must accept the mystery.
We must be a part of the mystery.
We must be encompassed by the mystery.

What is not mystery?

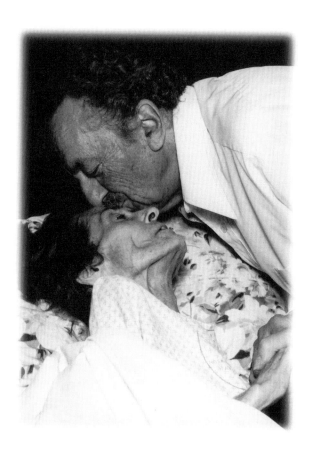

The strength of the caregiver
does not come from what he possesses.
The strength of the caregiver
comes from what possesses him.

Possessions are manifestations of being.
How one is possessed is the ground of being.
The caregiver rests in the ground of his being.

The caregiver is possessed by empathy.
The caregiver is possessed by compassion.
The caregiver is possessed by love.

Taking no credit,
the caregiver of the dying allows himself
to feel empathy, compassion, and love.
Taking no credit,
the caregiver of the dying then acts
with empathy, compassion, and love.

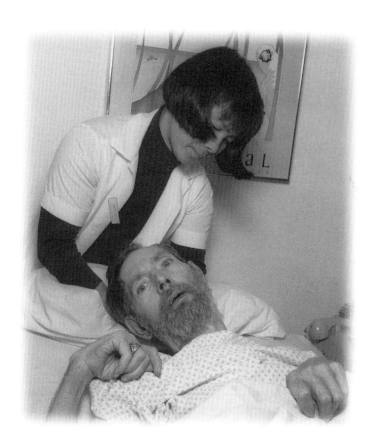

A good athlete allows her team to take the credit.
A good teacher allows her students
to feel their achievement.
A good boss allows her employees to receive the profit.
A good minister allows her congregation
to discover its god.

The dying need their caregivers.
The caregivers need their dying.

Only the fool claims to be without needs.

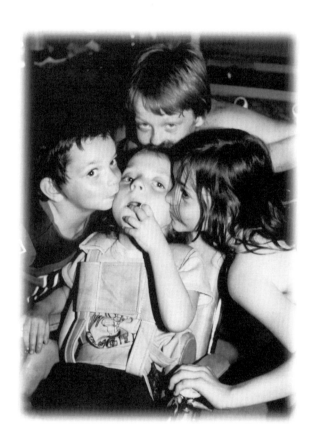

It is easy to take control.
It is good to not take control.

Grow through children.
Learn from students.
Live by receiving the dying.

Be like an uncarved block of wood.
Be like unmolded, pliable clay.
Be like unpainted, virgin canvas.
Allow the artist to have her joy.

Do you think that you can eliminate death?

Do you believe that you can postpone death?

Do you imagine you can even have the slightest effect on death?

Do not be fooled: we cannot control death.

Time is established.
It cannot be altered.
A year will always be a year.
A person's last year cannot be lengthened
or shortened.
A month will always be a month.
A person's last month cannot be lengthened
or shortened.
An hour will always be an hour.
A person's last hour cannot be lengthened
or shortened.

Do not reach forward.
Do not reach back.
Do not push.
Do not pull.
Be settled where you already are.

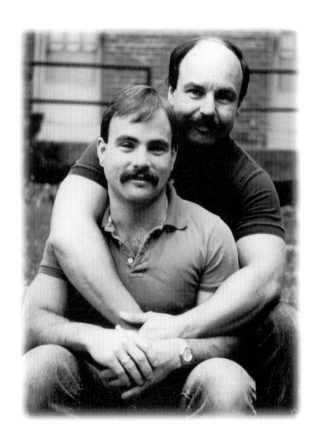

The caregiver does not invade another's space.
The caregiver does not exercise control.
The caregiver does not label.

The caregiver allows for the dying person's anger.
The caregiver allows for the dying person's depression.
The caregiver allows for the dying person's denial.

Styles of dying:
there are not good or bad ones.

In judging others,
the caregiver has judged himself
not worthy of giving care.
In not judging others,
the caregiver has judged himself
most worthy of giving care.

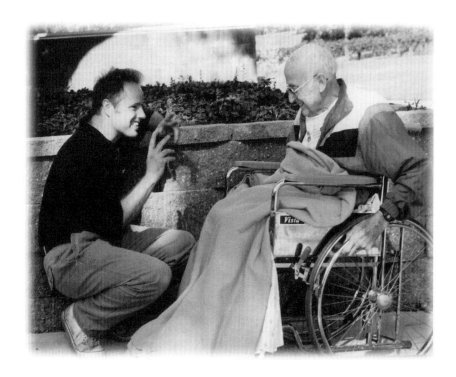

The caregiver refrains from asserting himself.
Asserting of self comes only after everything else fails.
Everything else fails only after everything else
has been tried.

Whenever the caregiver desires to assert himself,
he focuses upon his purpose in giving care.
Giving care means not pushing or pulling.
Giving care means not telling people
what they ought to do, think, or be.
Giving care means not trying to change people
who do not want to be changed.
Giving care means not trying to cure people
who cannot be cured.

Giving care means letting an individual be an individual.
Giving care means allowing, not controlling.
Giving care means receiving, not imposing.
Giving care means welcoming, not asserting.

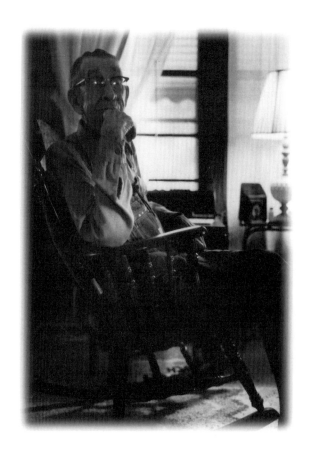

That which is most important does not have
to have beauty.
That which is most important does not have
to have strength.
That which is most important does not have
to have intelligence.
That which is most important arrives serendipitously.

Remember what is most important
and how it arrives,
and all will be peaceful,
and all will be right,
and all will be done.

Forget about philosophies and theories.
Forget about words and concepts.
Why limit yourself when you exist within the limitless?

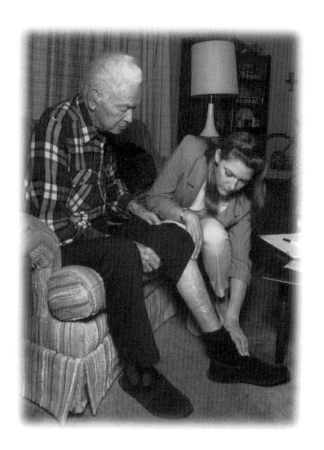

Accept life.

Accept death.

Can we really do anything else?

It is a mark of intelligence to know about others.

It is a mark of true enlightenment to know yourself.

It is a mark of strength to help others to move.

It is a mark of true power to get yourself to move.

It is a mark of richness to assist others
in finding contentment.

It is a mark of true wealth to get yourself to feel content.

Embrace your own death before it embraces you.

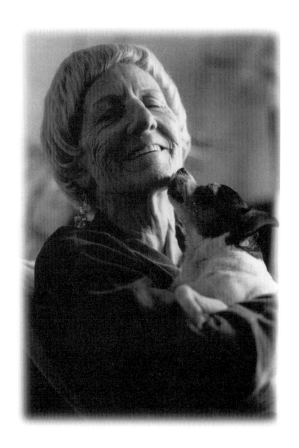

The mystery of life and death is found everywhere.
No one can escape the mystery of life and death.

So become absorbed in the mystery.
Let it play with you both day and night.

The mystery can be seen in a vast ocean.
Yet it can also be seen in a single tear.
It can be heard in a classical symphony.
Yet it can also be heard in a single sigh.
It can be felt through the applauding hands
of a great audience.
Yet it can also be felt through the touch of a single hand.

So the caregiver of the dying acknowledges the big,
yet concentrates on the small.

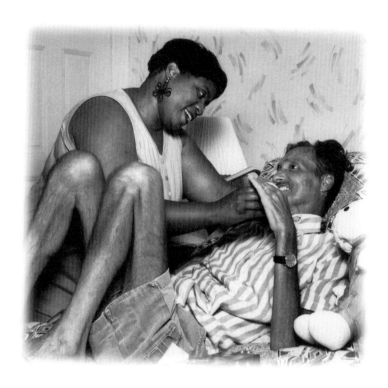

She who is absorbed in the mystery
has no desire to step out of the mystery.
She perceives the living and dying process
knowing that as she comforts others
her own comfort is found.

Onlookers will question her purpose.
Onlookers will question her pleasure.
What do they know who have not seen a single tear?
What do they know who have not heard a single sigh?
What do they know who have not felt the touch
of a single hand?

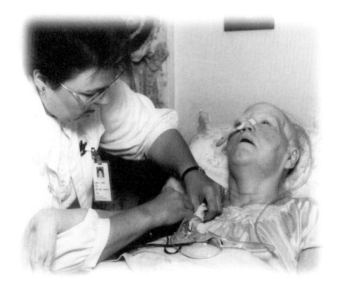

Flexibility makes no sense
   until you know the dangers of rigidity.
   Laughter seems so foolish
   until you know the dangers of seriousness.
   Touching is rarely considered
   until you know the dangers of distancing.
   Allowing has the appearance of uselessness
   until you know the dangers of controlling.

   The soft overpowers the hard.
   The slow outdistances the fast.

   Let those who question, question.
   Just do what needs to be done.

If we look at people as having problems,
problems will be what they experience.
If we look at people as having solutions,
solutions will be what they experience.
If we look at people as having weaknesses,
weaknesses will be what they experience.
If we look at people as having strengths,
strengths will be what they experience.

Putting yourself in the shadows
allows the other to experience the light.

By doing more,
less will be accomplished.
By doing less,
more will be accomplished.

The effective caregiver must confess
that he does nothing at all.

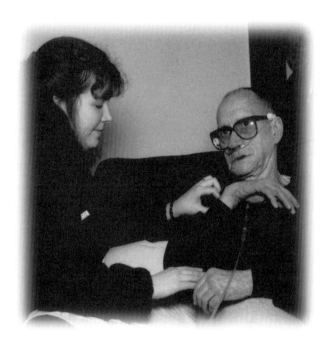

Giving credit where credit is due,
the caregiver will take no credit at all.
Thus, she shows love.

When the caregiver forgets some of the truth,
goodness will be shown.
When the caregiver forgets most of the truth,
morality will be shown.
When the caregiver forgets all of the truth,
propriety will be shown.

Propriety is totally a sham.
Morality is mostly a sham.
Goodness is partially a sham.
Love is no sham at all.

Shun propriety.
Avoid morality.
Be leery of goodness.
Embrace love.

Having no illusions,
the caregiver will take no credit at all.

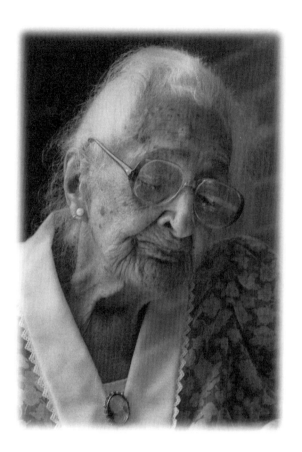

There can be significance in a dying person's elation.
There can be significance in a dying person's depression.
There can be significance in a dying person's composure.
There can be significance in a dying person's anxiety.
There can be significance in a dying person's acceptance.
There can be significance in a dying person's denial.

The caregiver knows
that there can be significance in everything.
She allows the dying to determine
what is most significant.

If the caregiver fights against elation,
or fights against depression,
or fights against composure,
or fights against anxiety,
or fights against acceptance,
or fights against denial,
she has destroyed what is significant.

As the caregiver enters the shadows,
she allows the dying to know the light.

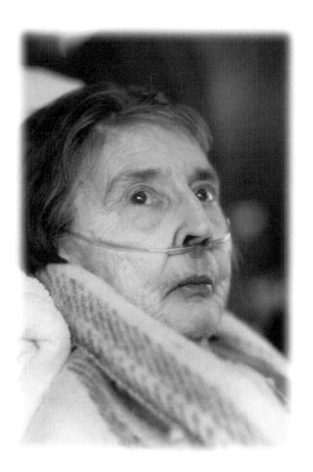

For a symphony to be beautiful,
there must be spaces between the notes.
Otherwise, there would only be a cacophony.

The dying will provide the notes.
The caregiver will provide the spaces.

Be attentive.
Listen.
Reflect.
Allow.

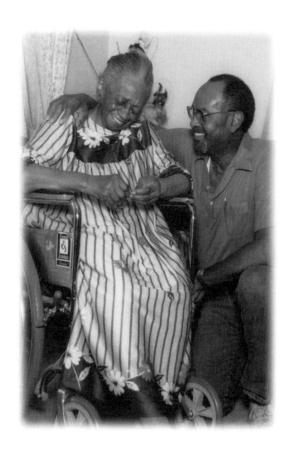

The superior caregiver allows for anything,
and all that needs to be accomplished is accomplished.
The average caregiver allows for some things,
and some of what needs to be accomplished
is accomplished.
The foolish caregiver (who is no caregiver at all)
needs to control everything,
and nothing is accomplished
that needs to be accomplished.

The superior caregiver sees life in the dying.
The foolish caregiver (who is no caregiver at all)
sees death in the dying.

Needs must be revealed before they can be met.
Do not control; do not assume.
Wants must be revealed before they can be met.
Do not control; do not assume.

Where is the superior caregiver?
Look in the shadows.

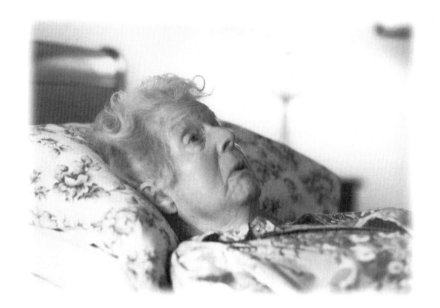

Show love toward one person,

    and it will seem like you are being loved by two,

    and it will feel like you are being loved by three,

    and it will be like you are being loved by everyone.

You are a half.

In loving the other, you are a whole.

In being whole, you rest in completeness.

Resting in completeness, all will be accomplished.

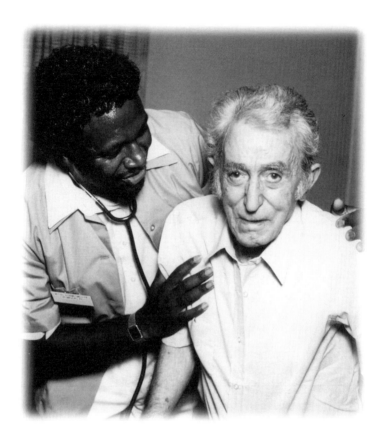

Being quiet can say more than a thousand words.
   Not having an imposing presence,
   the caregiver fits wherever needed.

   Speaking without saying anything at all,
   accomplishing without doing anything at all,
   the caregiver gives care.

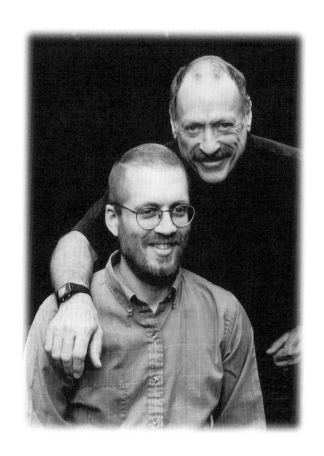

When the caregiver wants to control,
she experiences no control.
When the caregiver tries to gain,
she experiences no gain.
When the caregiver struggles to perpetuate life,
she experiences no life.

Allow.
Allow for loss.
Allow for the loss of life.

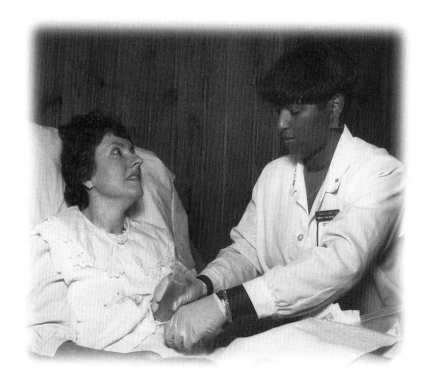

Stillness overcomes agitation.

Peace overcomes the warring emotions.

Simple truths confound the wisest intellect.

Laughter confounds the most serious of situations.

Why not be still?

Why not be at peace?

Why not be simple?

And never never forget to share the laughter!

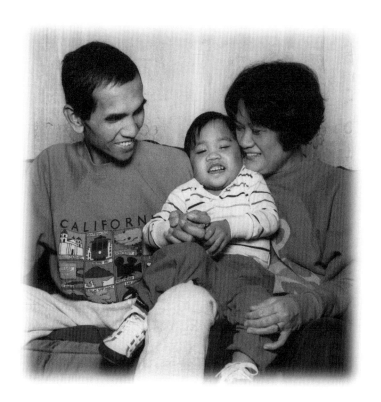

How unnaturally we usually treat the dying!
We treat them as already dead.
We put them in sterile environments.
We give them no attention.
We provide them with no touch.
We show them no laughter.

However, if we allow people to live until they die:
their environment is a living environment,
they can give and receive attention,
they can touch and be touched.

And never never forget to share the laughter!

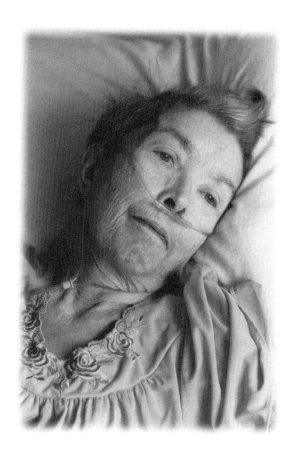

If you allow yourself to look within one person,
you can see the whole world.
If you allow yourself to receive one person,
you can receive the whole universe.

Yet if you try to look at the whole world,
you can see no one.
If you try to receive the whole universe,
you can receive no one.

The caregiver travels the universe without leaving home.
The caregiver accomplishes everything
without doing a thing.

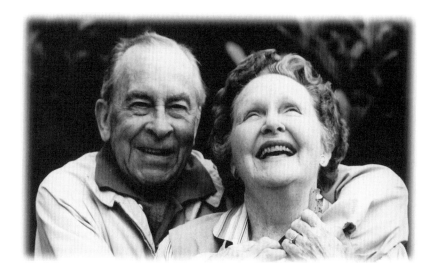

Those who do not know any better,
　　read about the latest theories and techniques.
　　In doing so, they fill their consciousness.
　　Thus, they have no room for the dying.

　　Those who know better
　　discard theories and techniques.
　　In doing so, they leave space in their consciousness.
　　Thus, they have some room for the dying.

　　The more space you have,
　　the more welcome the dying will feel.

　　Do not impose.
　　Simply repose.
　　Repose with open arms.

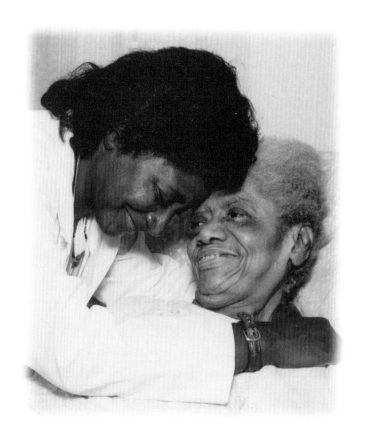

Without theories and techniques,
   the caregiver is like an empty vessel.
   Like an empty vessel,
   the caregiver's purpose is to receive.

   She trusts those who are worthy of trust.
   She trusts those who are not worthy of trust.
   She trusts without judging.

   She is good to those who are good.
   She is good to those who are not good.
   She possesses a nonjudgmental goodness.

   She loves those who earn her love.
   She loves those who do not earn her love.
   She loves without judging.

   The empty vessel does much by merely receiving.

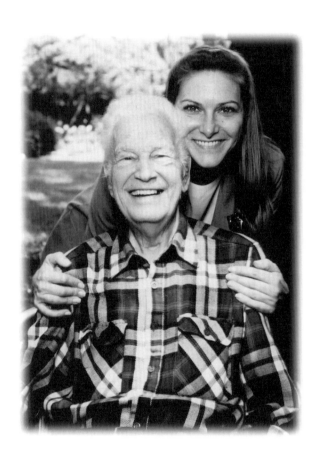

If you try to add to life,
   asking for more than what it gives,
   death will be seen as a robber,
   a robber that takes away all that you have.
   Yet if you receive life for what it naturally gives,
   dying will give you even more.

   The caregiver does not try to light fires
   where no fires are wanted.
   The caregiver does not rush to put out fires
   that never burn.

   The caregiver does not seek to give directions
   to someone who does not feel lost.

Every person in the universe
   is a manifestation of what is sacred.

   What is sacred?
   It cannot be grasped.
   Yet it can take hold.
   It cannot be pushed or pulled.
   Yet it can move you.
   It cannot be taught.
   Yet it can be learned.
   It cannot be controlled.
   Yet it can be allowed.

In listening to the voice of another,
the sacred is being revealed.
In accepting the hand of another,
the sacred is being revealed.

In allowing yourself to receive another,
the sacred is being revealed.

The sacred is not given.
The sacred is received.

So, do not impose your spirituality.
You have nothing to give.

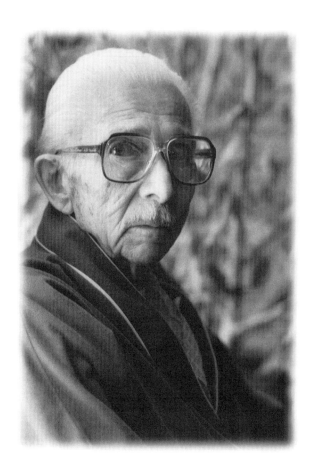

In the beginning there was life and death.
In the beginning there was right and wrong.
In the beginning there was beauty and ugliness.
In the beginning there was good and bad.

What is life without death?
What is right without wrong?
What is beauty without ugliness?
What is good without bad?

What makes you think that all can be life?
What makes you think that all can be right?
What makes you think that all can be beautiful?
What makes you think that all can be good?

Living is the process of leaving home.
Dying is the process of coming home.

The caregiver is at home
in allowing people to come and go.

Death can be very painful.
Do not waver in your attitude of allowing.

Death can be very exhausting.
Do not waver in your attitude of allowing.

Death can be very ugly.
Do not waver in your attitude of allowing.

Childbirth can be very painful, exhausting, and ugly.
Yet a beautiful child can still be born.
So it is with dying.

Do not judge the death by the dying!
Do not judge the dying!
Do not judge the death!
Do not judge!

Be prepared for anything.
Allow for anything.
Accept anything.

There is no other way.

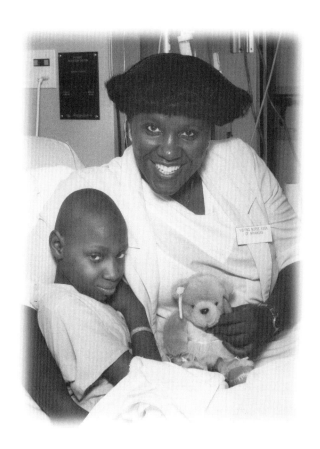

How can you accept another
if you cannot accept yourself?
How can you accept yourself
if you do not accept both the right and the wrong,
the beautiful and the ugly,
the good and the bad?

Accept yourself,
and you will learn how to accept another.
Accept another,
and you will learn how to accept a community.
Accept a community,
and you will learn how to accept a nation.
Accept a nation,
and you will learn how to accept the world.

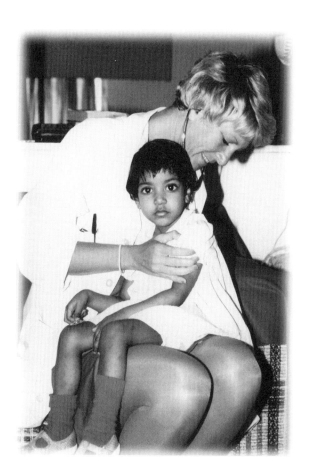

Not hardened, but as pliable as a child,
the caregiver allows.
Not closed, but as receptive as a child,
the caregiver allows.

Energy waiting to be directed: the caregiver awaits.
Energy waiting to be channeled: the caregiver awaits.
Energy waiting to be used: the caregiver awaits.
Energy waiting to be spent: the caregiver awaits.

Energy being spent: the caregiver takes no credit at all.

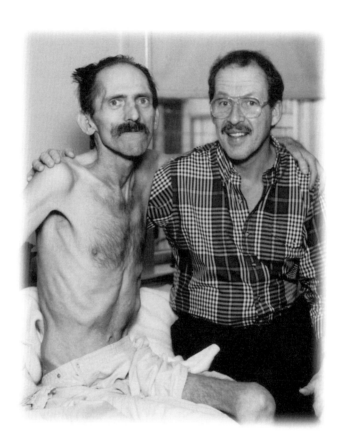

Those who perceive the universe as it is
are not verbose.
Those who are verbose
do not perceive the universe as it is.

Stop.

The caregiver stops his wandering thoughts
and becomes settled in his place.
The caregiver stops his wandering actions
and becomes settled in his place.

In quieting his mind,
the caregiver hears.
In restraining his body,
the caregiver accomplishes.

In denying himself,
the caregiver affirms the world.

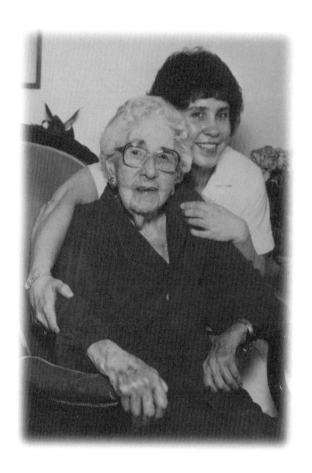

When philosophies abound, nothing is certain.
When guidelines are numerous, many are broken.

The caregiver cannot lose at a game he does not play.

Stop playing the game of control.
Nobody wants to play by your rules.
Everyone will always create their own rules.

Let go of trying to change the world
and the world, on its own, will change for the better.

The caregiver will see this truth revealed:
the world progresses when no one is pushing or pulling.

When we push or pull the world,
the world regresses.

Allow.

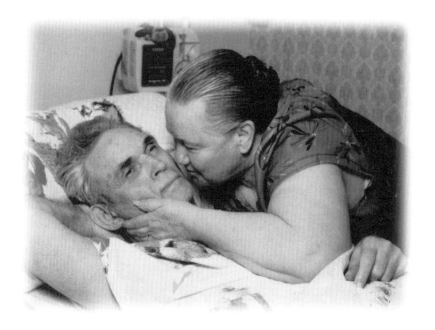

If there is anxiety,

let it reign.

A calm successor will eventually arrive.

If there is anger,

let it reign.

A peaceful successor will eventually arrive.

If there is denial,

let it reign.

The truth, of its own accord,

eventually makes itself known.

Every steadfast witness

experiences resolution.

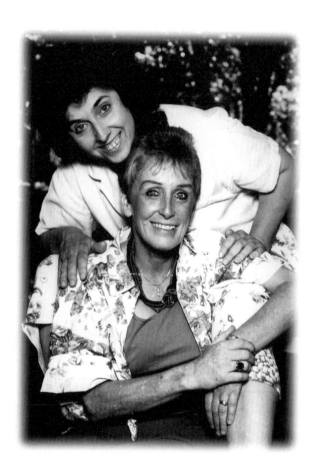

Be like everyone else
and you will be like everyone else.

Knowing how you are like everyone else
is the ultimate in knowledge.
When you gain this knowledge,
you have no need to try to be extraordinary.
You already are.

The caregiver does not strive,
because she realizes that she has already arrived.

In listening to another,
in holding hands with another,
in being with another,
the caregiver needs to be no place other than where she is.
She realizes that she has arrived before ever leaving.

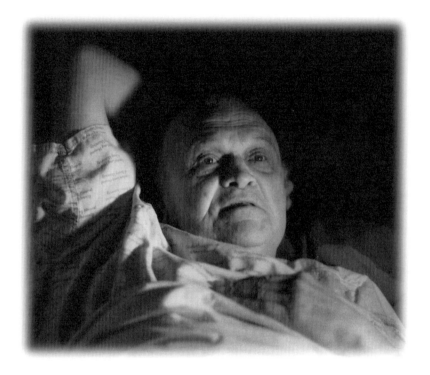

That which is not disturbed
cannot be defiled.
That which is not attacked
cannot be violated.

Allowing people to be who they are
allows them to be who they want to be.

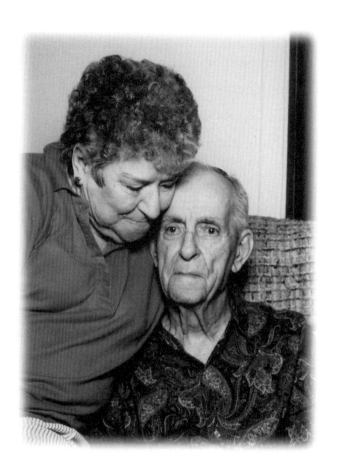

The sea is mightier than any river.
Yet the sea lies below any river,
is open to any river,
and receives any river.

The caregiver of the dying represents a sea of love.

There might be an angry, rushing river.
There might be a lazy, tired river.
There might be a crooked, treacherous river.
There might be a polluted river.
The sea is open to them all.
The sea receives them all.
They are all transformed in the sea
because the sea allows them to transform.

The caregiver of the dying represents a sea of love.

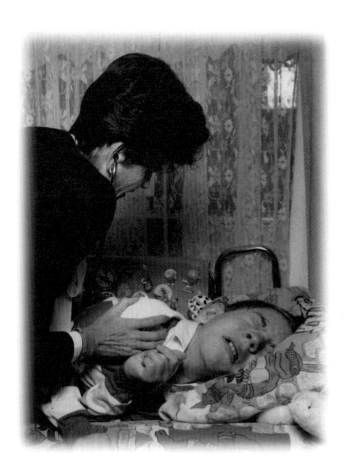

Impartiality is a type of allowing.

So is forgiveness.

So is compassion.

So is love.

The caregiver reveals impartiality.

She shows forgiveness.

She announces compassion.

She shouts love.

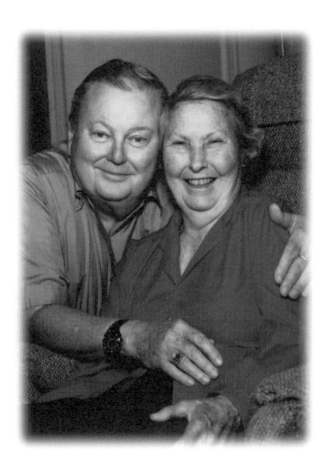

Accomplish many things without doing anything.
Find value in what others consider worthless.
Attain heights where others perceive only depths.

Envision the insignificant as great.
Ascertain that the small is really quite large.
Return gentleness when harshly attacked.
Answer with kindness when questioned with anger.

That which has value
always begins as something with no worth.
That which is great
always arises from that which has no significance.

When the caregiver is confronted with a challenge,
he receives it without hesitating.
He does not worry about his own welfare.
So nothing can be a problem for him.

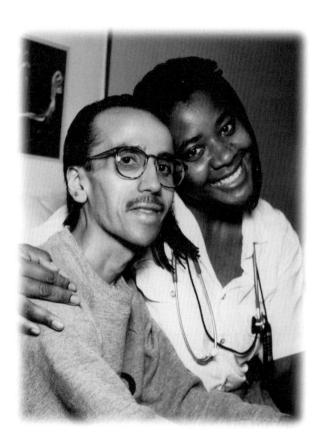

Be patient.
Those who are too eager
lose their ability to be present.
The caregiver maintains presence.

Be calm.
Those who are too agitated
lose their balance.
The caregiver maintains balance.

Be loving.
Those who are too concerned about themselves
lose everything else.
The caregiver opens herself to receive all.

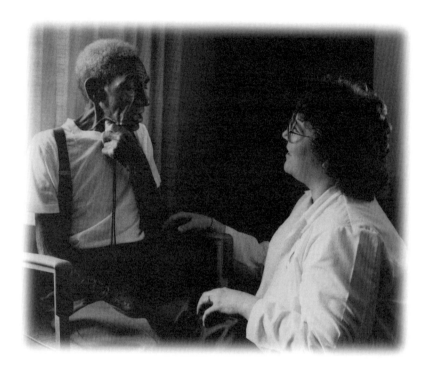

The caregiver believes she has no advantages
   over the dying person
   and therefore becomes quite advantageous
   to the dying person.

If the caregiver is content with little things,
   she has no need to seek greater things.
   If the caregiver is satisfied with simple pleasures,
   she can ignore pleasures that are beyond reach.

In seeking to master the art of direction,
   the caregiver follows directions quite well.
   In seeking to master leadership,
   the caregiver masters the art of following.

Who is the perfect caregiver?
   It is the caregiver who feels the furthest from perfection.

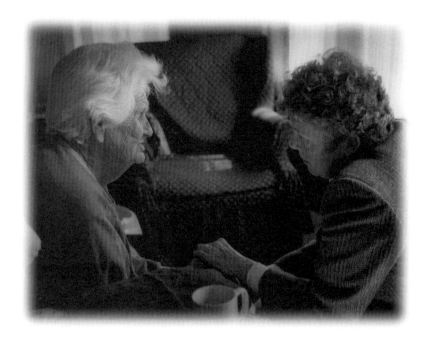

Because the caregiver has the attitude of allowing,
   she cannot be surprised by anything.
   Nothing catches her unprepared.
   Nothing is too great for her.
   Nothing is too small for her.

   The caregiver has more capabilities than the dying.
   Yet the dying feel no envy.

   By accepting,
   the caregiver is accepted.
   By not judging,
   the caregiver is judged trustworthy.

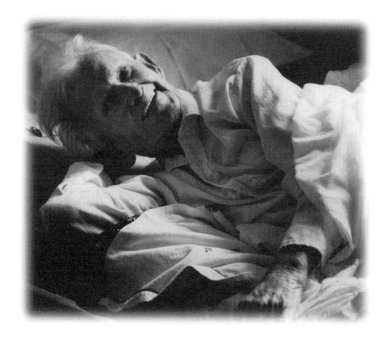

People say that it is absurd to allow the dying
to have control.
People say that such an idea is impractical.

Look inside yourself.

Would you feel comfort around the person
who gives you choices or the person who takes choices
away from you?
Would you respect the person who trusts your decisions
or the person who does not allow you to make decisions?

Would you cheat a marathon runner out of his last mile?
Would you take the brush away from an artist
before he makes his signature?

The caregiver has the attitude of allowing.
That is the greatest wisdom.
That is being very practical.

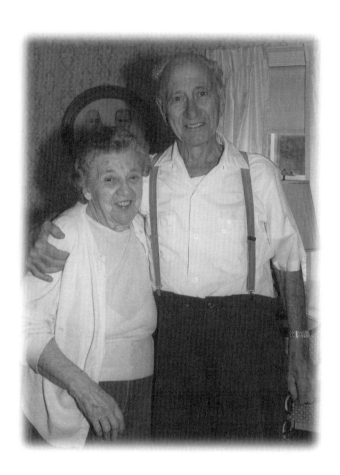

Is not life given to everyone?

Is not life taken away from everyone?

Does not everyone get exactly one life?

Does any individual get more than one life?

Does any individual get less than one life?

Can anyone have one life plus an hour?

Can anyone have one life minus an hour?

Why all the complaining?

Why all the struggling?

Why all the competition?

Accept your life.

Accept the lives of others.

What if complaining, struggling, and competition
were replaced by tolerance, love, and play?

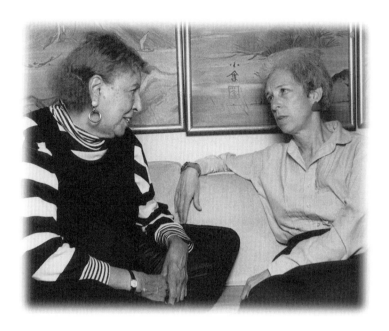

If aggression has an opponent,
   aggression is fueled.
   With no opponent,
   aggression runs a limited course
   and then expires.

   If anger has an opponent,
   anger is fueled.
   With no opponent,
   anger runs a limited course
   and then expires.

   Aggression and anger will always be around.
   Yet, by allowing them to exist,
   their course becomes limited.

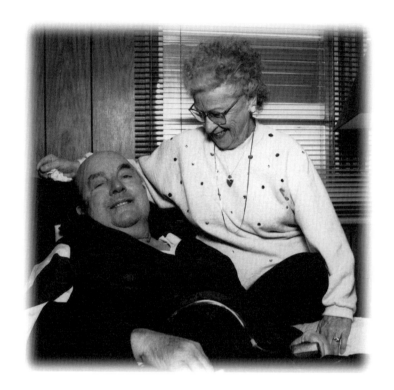

The caregiver's task is easy to describe
and easy to practice.
Yet people continually make it difficult.

There is much we need to unlearn.
There is much we need to not express.
There is much we need to not do.

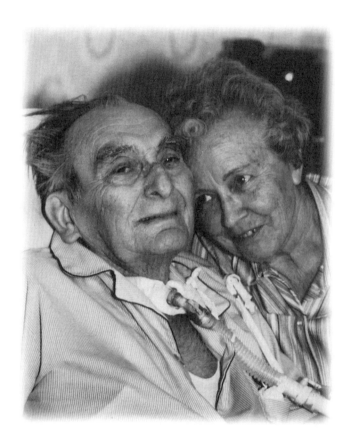

A good learner has humility.
A good teacher has humility.

Humility marks a good giver.
Humility marks a good receiver.

A good follower has humility.
A good leader has humility.

Humility: an indispensable ingredient in living.
Humility: an indispensable ingredient in dying.

The caregiver knows all about humility.

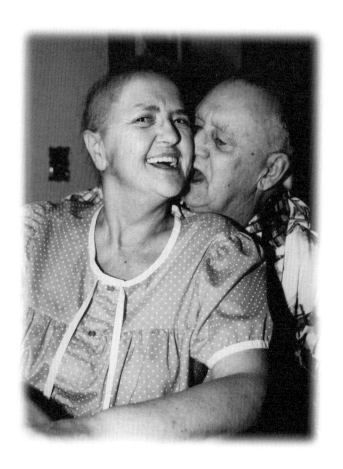

To allow is to yield.
To yield is to produce.

In allowing, the caregiver produces much.
Yet the caregiver deserves no credit
since he is merely yielding to something greater.

Listen to that which speaks for itself!
Do not confuse by talking.
Do not disrupt by doing.
Allow by yielding.
Produce by yielding.

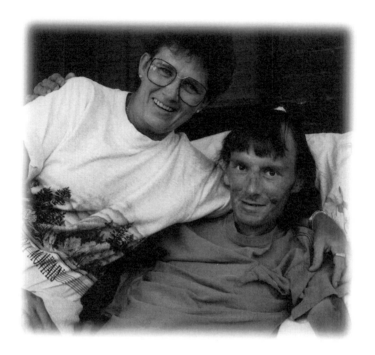

Without preaching a sermon
   or making moral demands,
   the caregiver represents what is holy.

Allowing for freedom can have divine results.
Giving people choices is a sacred calling.

Encircling her arms around one person,
the caregiver encompasses the whole world.

Thus, the caregiver knows humility.
Thus, the caregiver knows godliness.

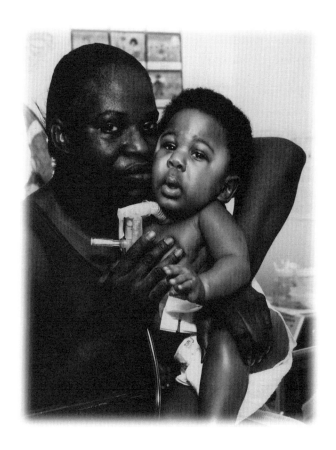

In realizing that everything changes,
the caregiver has no need to hold onto anything.
The caregiver seeks to master the art of letting go.

In working with the dying,
the caregiver needs to know how to die.
To know how to die,
the caregiver has to let go of control:
letting go of the past,
letting go of the present,
letting go of the future.

After letting go of everything she has,
the caregiver has unlimited potential.

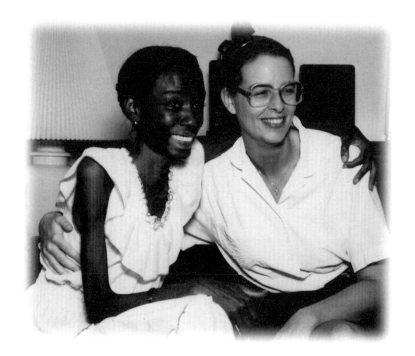

Respect other people as much as you respect yourself,
for they are just as worthy of respect as you.
Trust other people as much as you trust yourself,
for they are just as worthy of trust as you.
Love other people as much as you love yourself,
for they are just as worthy of love as you.

Things will upset you.
You will suffer.
You will question the value of life.
Yet remember two things:
You are not alone.
You need to love and be loved.

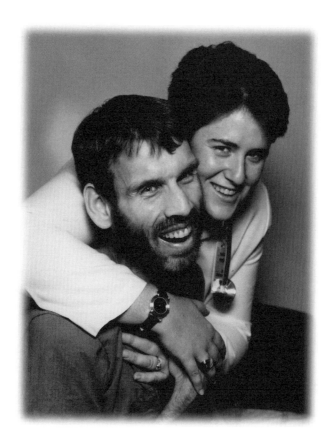

When heavy winds come,

the oak tree's branches break and fall to the ground.

The oak is stiff and unyielding.

The willow bends and springs back to life and wholeness.

When heavy rains come,

the maple tree's branches break and fall to the ground.

The maple is stiff and unyielding.

The willow bends and springs back to life and wholeness.

When heavy snows come,

the pine tree's branches break and fall to the ground.

The pine is stiff and unyielding.

The willow bends and springs back to life and wholeness.

The caregiver of the dying bends and springs back

to life and wholeness.

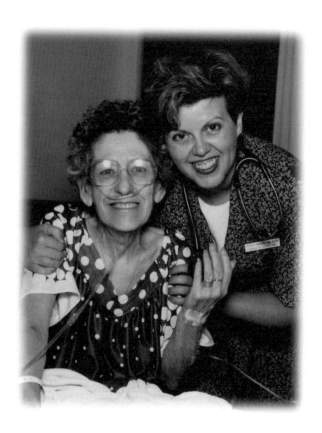

Coming without expectations,
the caregiver feels no disappointment.
Coming without the need to experience success,
the caregiver feels no failure.
Coming without the need to exercise power,
the caregiver feels no weaknesses.

Without trying to take,
the caregiver receives in multiple ways.

Trying to control is fruitless.
Yet a rich harvest comes to those who allow for growth.

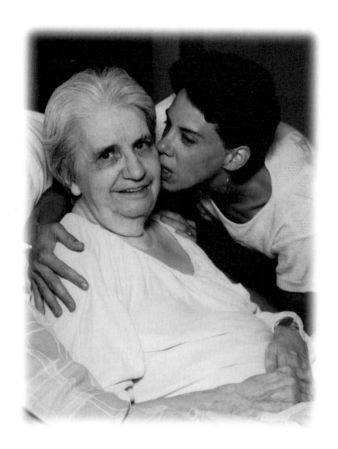

Who is the one who rests in the eye of a storm?
Who is the one who can find refreshing streams
in the middle of a desert?
Who is the one who can see clearly at the darkest hour?

Is there anything greater and more powerful
than peace and contentment?

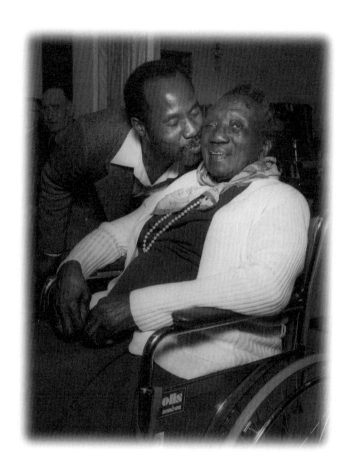

For the caregiver,
pain presents an opportunity,
an opportunity for witnessing the relief of pain.

For the caregiver,
anxiety presents an opportunity,
an opportunity for witnessing the development of calm.

For the caregiver,
anger presents an opportunity,
an opportunity for witnessing the establishment of peace.

For the caregiver,
dying presents an opportunity,
an opportunity for witnessing the discovery of life.

The caregiver does not demand anything.
Yet he receives many opportunities.

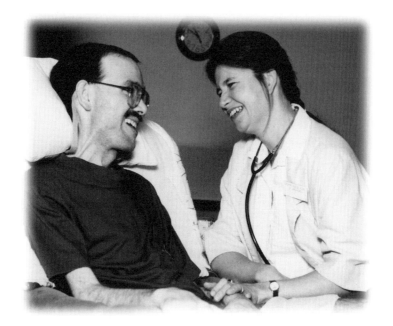

The dying can look at the caregiver and see themselves.
The dying can listen to the caregiver and hear themselves.

The value of the caregiver is found
in the self-worth of the dying.

The dying feel empowered
within the presence of the caregiver.

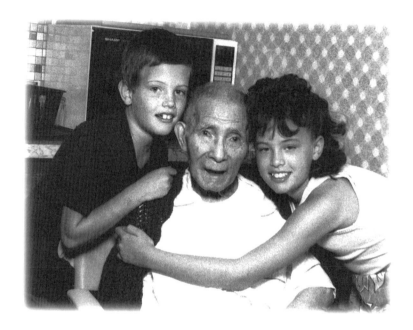

In letting go,
  there is gain.
  In giving up,
  there is advancement.

Do not practice controlling.
Practice allowing.

Such is the mystery of happiness.
Such is the mystery of wealth.
Such is the mystery of power.
Such is the mystery of living and dying.

Douglas C. Smith

Doug is the Senior Associate of Operations at the Hospice of Central Iowa. He also presents workshops on patient care for hospices around the country. Doug brings to those workshops, to the work at Hospice of Central Iowa, and to this book a holistic perspective that comes from having master's degrees in three different disciplines: an MDiv from the Protestant Episcopal Theological Seminary in Virginia; an MA from Bradley University, and an MS from California College for Health Sciences. He has been published in *CARING* Magazine, *Counseling and Values*, *The Journal of Humanistic Education and Development*, *Omega: Journal of Death and Dying*, *The Hospice Journal*, *The American Journal of Hospice & Palliative Care*, *Illness, Crisis and Loss*, *The Medical Hypnoanalysis Journal*, and *The Journal for Specialists in Group Work*. Much of his writing, including this book, has centered around two concepts that he has been researching: healthy death and psychopalliation. Both concepts address the question, "How is it possible to die in an environment that allows the dying person to have respect, dignity, and as much control as possible?"

Marilu Pittman

Marilu Pittman has been photographing hospice and home care patients for more than 12 years. She has traveled throughout the country, documenting the courage of the terminally ill and the compassion of those who care for them. Her photographs are featured prominently in *CARING* Magazine, the national monthly magazine of the National Association for Home Care. Her photographs are also found in *Caring People* magazine, a national quarterly magazine dedicated to celebrating the human spirit and the importance of service to others. Her work has been highlighted in both national and international publications, including *PARADE* magazine, *Modern Maturity*, *World Health*, *Nursing & Health Care*, *Generations*, *In-depth Views of Issues in Aging*, *Geriatric Nursing*, and *American Journal of Care for the Aging*. Her photographs have appeared in books as well, including *Health Care: Careers for Today* (visual Education Corp., 1991), *Profiles in Caring: Advocates for the Elderly* (Caring Publishing, 1991), and *Faces of Caring: A Search for the 100 Most Caring People in History* (Caring Publishing, 1992).